Dash Diet Delicacies

The Definitive Super Tasty Collection for your
everyday Dash Diet Meals

Natalie Puckett

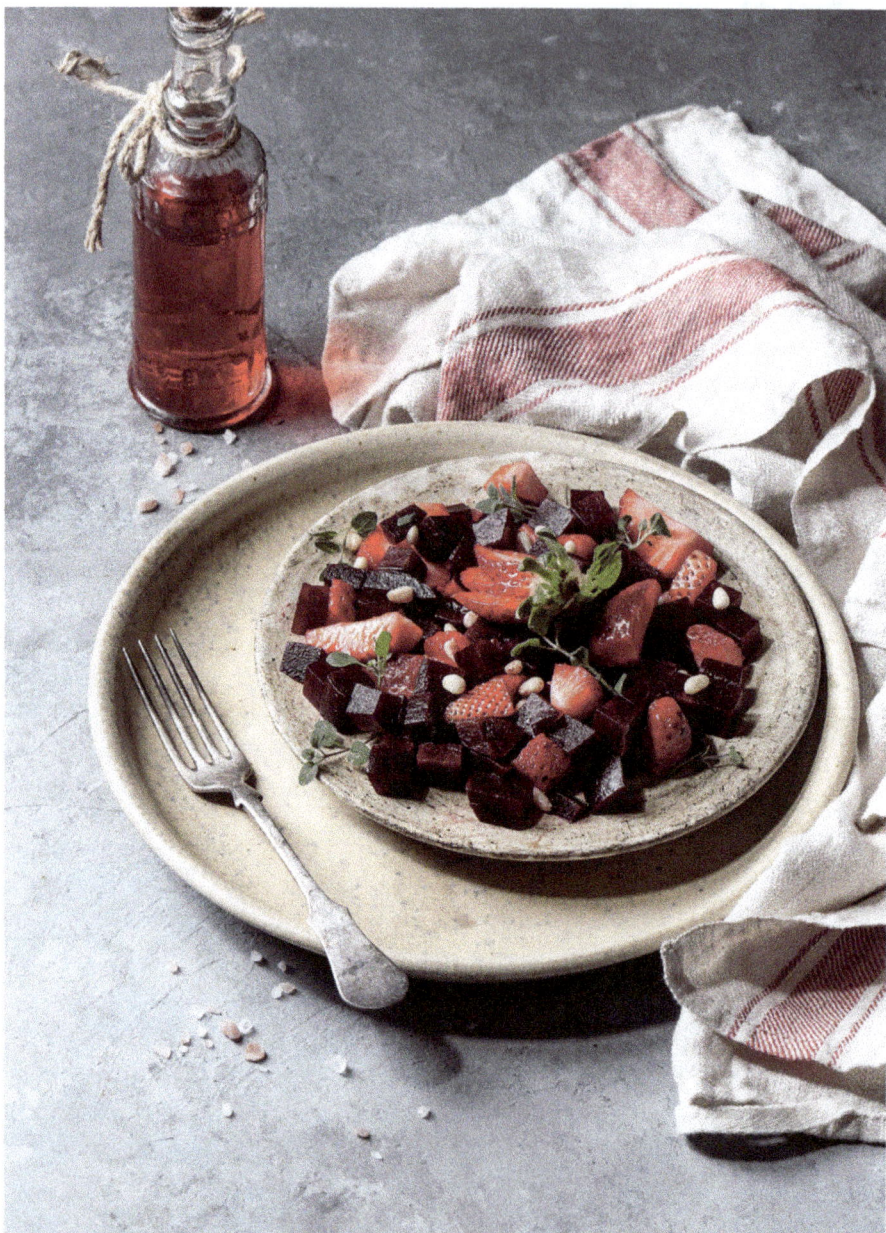

Table of Contents

Pork and Balsamic Strawberry Salad

Ingredients

One pork tenderloin (1 pound)

1/2 cup Italian salad dressing

1-1/2 cups halved fresh strawberries

Two tablespoons balsamic vinegar

Two teaspoons sugar

1/4 teaspoon salt

1/4 teaspoon pepper

Two tablespoons olive oil

1/4 cup chicken broth

One package about 5 ounces spring mix salad greens 1/2 cup crumbled goat cheese

Instructions

1.   Place pork during a shallow dish. Add salad dressing; flip for coating. Refrigerate and canopy for a minimum of eight hours. Mix strawberries, vinegar and sugar; cover and refrigerate.

2.   Preheat oven to 425°. Drain and wipe off meat , discarding marinade. Sprinkle with salt and pepper. during a large cast-iron or every other ovenproof skillet, warmness oil over medium-high warmness. Add beef; brown on all sides.

3.   Bake until a thermometer reads 145°, 15-20 minutes. Remove from skillet; permit or stand 5 min. Then, add broth to skillet; cook over medium warmth, stirring to loosen browned bits from pan. bring back a boil. Reduce warmth; add strawberry. Then heat it.

4.   Place green vegetables on a serving platter; sprinkle with cheese. Slice pork; found out over veggies. Top with strawberry mixture.

Nutrition

291 calories, 16g fat (5g saturated fat), 81mg cholesterol, 444mg sodium, 12g carbohydrate (7g sugars, 3g fibre), 26g protein.

Peppered Tuna Kabobs

Ingredients

1/2 cup frozen corn, thawed Four green onions, chopped One jalapeno pepper, seeded and chopped

Two tablespoons coarsely chopped fresh parsley Two tablespoons lime juice

1 pound tuna steaks, cut into 1-inch cubes One teaspoon coarsely ground pepper

Two large sweet red peppers, cut into 2x1-inch pieces

Instructions

1.   One medium mango, peeled and cut into 1-inch cubes

2.   For salsa, during a small bowl, combine the primary five ingredients; put aside.

3.   Rub tuna with pepper. On 4metal or soaked wooden skewers, alternately thread red peppers, tuna and mango.

4.   Place skewers on greased grill rack. Cook, covered, over medium heat, occasionally turning, until tuna is slightly pink in centre (medium-rare) and peppers are tender 10-12 minutes. Serve with salsa.

Nutrition

205 calories, 2g fat (0 saturated fat), 51mg cholesterol, 50mg sodium, 20g carbohydrate (12g sugars, 4g fibre), 29g protein

Weeknight Chicken Chop Suey

Ingredients

Four teaspoons of olive oil

1 pound of boneless chicken breast side, cut into 1-inch cubes

1/2 teaspoon dried tarragon

1/2 teaspoon dried basil

1/2 teaspoon dried marjoram

1/2 teaspoon grated lemon zest

1-1/2 cups chopped carrots

1 cup unsweetened pineapple tidbits, drained (reserve juice)

One can (8 ounces) sliced water chestnuts, drained

One medium tart apple, chopped

1/2 cup chopped onion

1 cup cold water, divided

Three tablespoons unsweetened pineapple juice

Three tablespoons reduced-sodium teriyaki sauce

Two tablespoons cornstarch

3 cups hot cooked brown rice

Instructions

1.   In a massive cast-iron or another heavy skillet, heat oil at medium temperature. Add chicken, herbs and lemon zest; leave it until lightly browned. Add subsequent five ingredients. Stir in 3/four cup water, fruit juice and teriyaki sauce; bring back a boil. Reduce warmness; simmer covered till chicken is not any longer purple, and therefore the carrots are gentle 10-15 minutes.

2.   Combine cornstarch and remaining water. Gradually stir into hen mixture. Leave for boiling; cook and stir till thickened, about 2 minutes. Serve with rice.

Nutrition

330 calories, 6g fat, 42mg cholesterol, 227mg sodium, 50g carbohydrate (14g sugars, 5g fibre), 20g protein

Thai Chicken Pasta Skillet

Ingredients

6 ounces uncooked whole-wheat spaghetti Two teaspoons canola oil

One package (10 ounces) fresh sugar snap peas, trimmed and cut diagonally into thin strips

2 cups julienned carrots (about 8 ounces)

2 cups shredded cooked chicken

1 cup Thai peanut sauce

One medium cucumber, halved lengthwise, seeded and sliced diagonally

Chopped fresh cilantro, optional

Instructions

1.	Cook spaghetti according to package directions; drain.

2.	Then, during a large skillet, heat oil a medium-high heat. Add snap peas and carrots; stir-fry 6-8 minutes or until crisp tender. Add chicken, peanut sauce and spaghetti; heat through, tossing to mix.

3.	Transfer to a serving plate. Top with cucumber and, if desired, cilantro.

Nutrition Facts

403 calories, 15g fat (3g saturated fat), 42mg cholesterol, 432mg sodium, 43g carbohydrate (15g sugars, 6g fibre), 25g protein

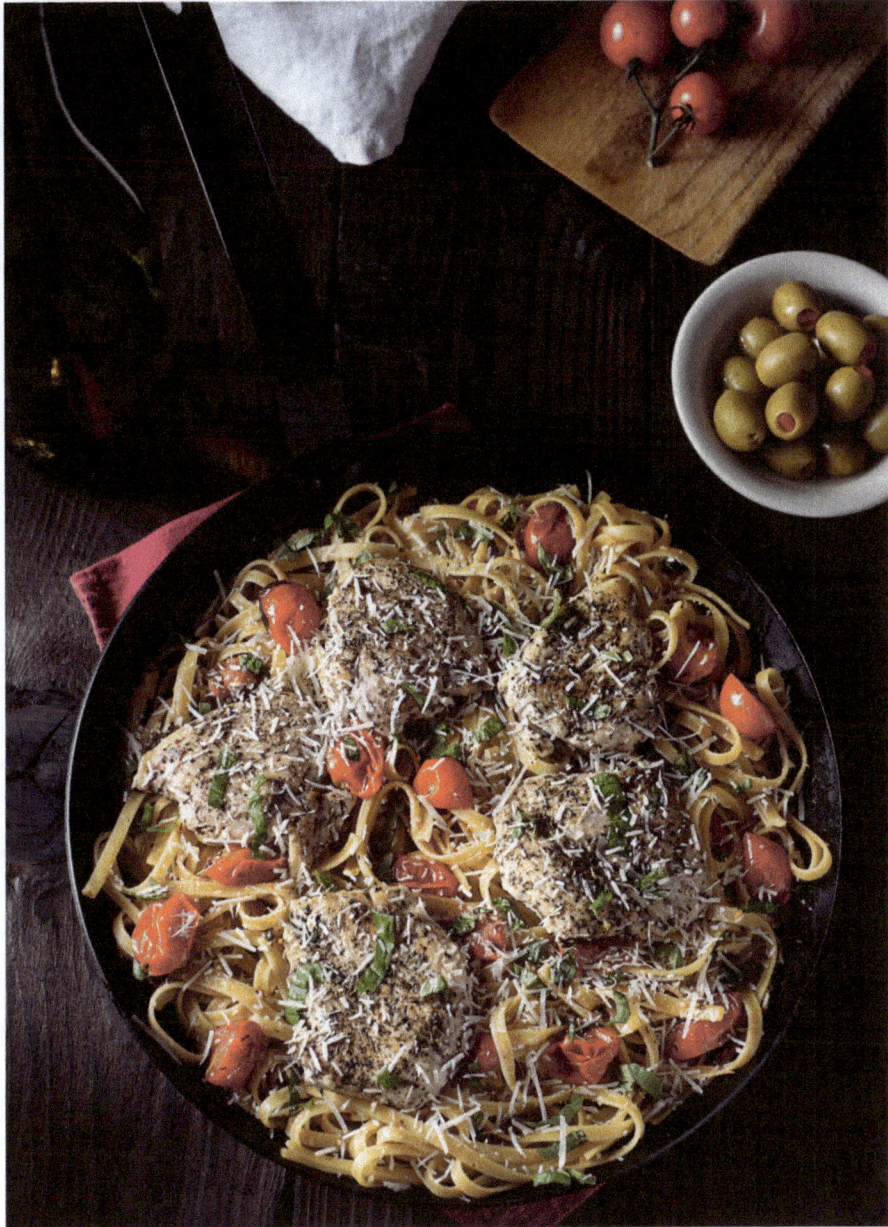

Spinach-Orzo Salad with Chickpeas

Ingredients

One 14-1/2 ounces reduced-sodium chicken broth 1-1/2 cups of uncooked whole wheat orzo pasta 4 cups of fresh baby spinach

2 cups of grape tomatoes, halved

Two cans (15 ounces each) of chickpeas or garbanzo beans, rinsed and drained

3/4 cup chopped fresh parsley

Two green onions, chopped

DRESSING:

1/4 cup olive oil

Three tablespoons lemon juice

3/4 teaspoon salt

1/4 teaspoon garlic powder

1/4 teaspoon hot pepper sauce

1/4 teaspoon pepper

Instructions

1.   Take an outsized saucepan and convey broth to a boil. Stir in orzo; return to a boil. Reduce heat; simmer, covered, until hard, 8-10 minutes.

2.   Take an outsized pan and add spinach and warm orzo, allowing the spinach to wilt slightly. Add tomatoes, chickpeas, parsley and green onions.

3.   Whisk together dressing ingredients. Toss with salad.

Nutrition

122 calories, 5g fat, 0 cholesterol, 259mg sodium, 16g carbohydrate (1g sugars, 4g fibre), 4g protein. Diabetic Exchanges: 1 starch, one fat.

Roasted Chicken Thighs with Peppers & Potatoes

Ingredients

2 pounds red potatoes (about six medium)

Two large sweet red peppers

Two large green peppers

Two medium onions

Two tablespoons olive oil, divided

Four teaspoons minced fresh thyme or 1-1/2 teaspoons dried thyme, divided

Three teaspoons minced fresh rosemary or one teaspoon dried rosemary, crushed, divided

Eight boneless skinless chicken thighs (about 2 pounds)

1/2 teaspoon salt

1/4 teaspoon pepper

Instructions

1.   Preheat oven to 450°. Cut potatoes, peppers and onions into 1-in. Pieces. Place vegetables during a roasting pan. Drizzle with one tablespoon oil; sprinkle with two teaspoons each thyme and rosemary and toss to coat. Place chicken over greens. Brush

chicken with remaining oil; sprinkle with remaining thyme and rosemary. Drizzle vegetables and chicken with salt and pepper.

2.   Roast until a thermometer inserted in chicken reads 170° and green vegetables are tender 35-40 minutes.

Nutrition Facts

308 calories, 12g fat (3g saturated fat), 76mg cholesterol, 221mg sodium, 25g carbohydrate (5g sugars, 4g fibre), 24g protein. Diabetic Exchanges: 3 lean meat, one starch, one vegetable, 1/2 fat.

Spiced Split Pea Soup

Ingredients

1 cup dried green split peas

Two medium potatoes, chopped

Two medium carrots, halved and thinly sliced

One medium onion, chopped

One celery rib, thinly sliced

Three garlic cloves, minced

Three bay leaves

Four teaspoons curry powder

One teaspoon ground cumin

1/2 teaspoon coarsely ground pepper

1/2 teaspoon ground coriander

One carton (32 ounces) reduced-sodium chicken broth One can (28 ounces) diced tomatoes, undrained

Instructions

1.   In a 4-qt. Slow cooker combines the primary 12 ingredients. Cook, covered, on low until peas are tender, 8-10 hours.

2.   Stir in tomatoes; heat through. Discard bay leaves.

Nutrition Facts

139 calories, 0 fat (0 saturated fat), 0 cholesterol, 347mg sodium, 27g carbohydrate (7g sugars, 8g fibre), 8g protein. Diabetic Exchanges: 1 starch, one lean meat, one vegetable.

Escarole and Bean Soup

Ingredients

Two tablespoons olive oil

Two chopped garlic cloves

1 pound of escarole, chopped

Salt

4 cups of low-salt broth chicken

1 can of cannellini bean

1 (1-ounce) piece of Parmesan

Freshly ground black pepper

Six teaspoons extra-virgin olive oil

Directions

1.   Heat vegetable oil during a big heavy pot at normal heat. Add the garlic and sauté till fragrant, for 15 seconds. Add the escarole and sauté till wilted, for 2 min. Add salt. Add the chicken, beans, then Parmesan cheese. Cover and simmer till the beans are heated through, approximately five minutes — season with salt and pepper, to taste.

2.   Ladle the soup into six bowls. Sprinkle one teaspoon extra-virgin vegetable oil over each. Serve with crusty bread.

Creamy Shrimp Salad

Serving: 4

Prep Time: 20 minutes

Cook Time: 5 minutes

Ingredients:

4 pounds large shrimp

1 lemon, quartered

3 cups celery stalks, chopped

1 red onion, chopped

2 cups mayonnaise

2 tablespoons white wine vinegar

1 teaspoon Dijon mustard

Salt and pepper as needed

How To:

1.   Take a large pan and place it over medium heat.

2.   Add water (salted) and bring water to boil.

3.   Add shrimp and lemon, cook for 3 minutes.

4.   Let them cool.

5.   Peel and de-vein the shrimps.

6.   Take a large bowl and add cooked shrimp alongside remaining ingredients.

7.   Stir well.

8.   Serve immediately or chilled!

Nutrition (Per Serving)

Calories: 153

Fat: 5g

Carbohydrates: 8g

Protein: 19g

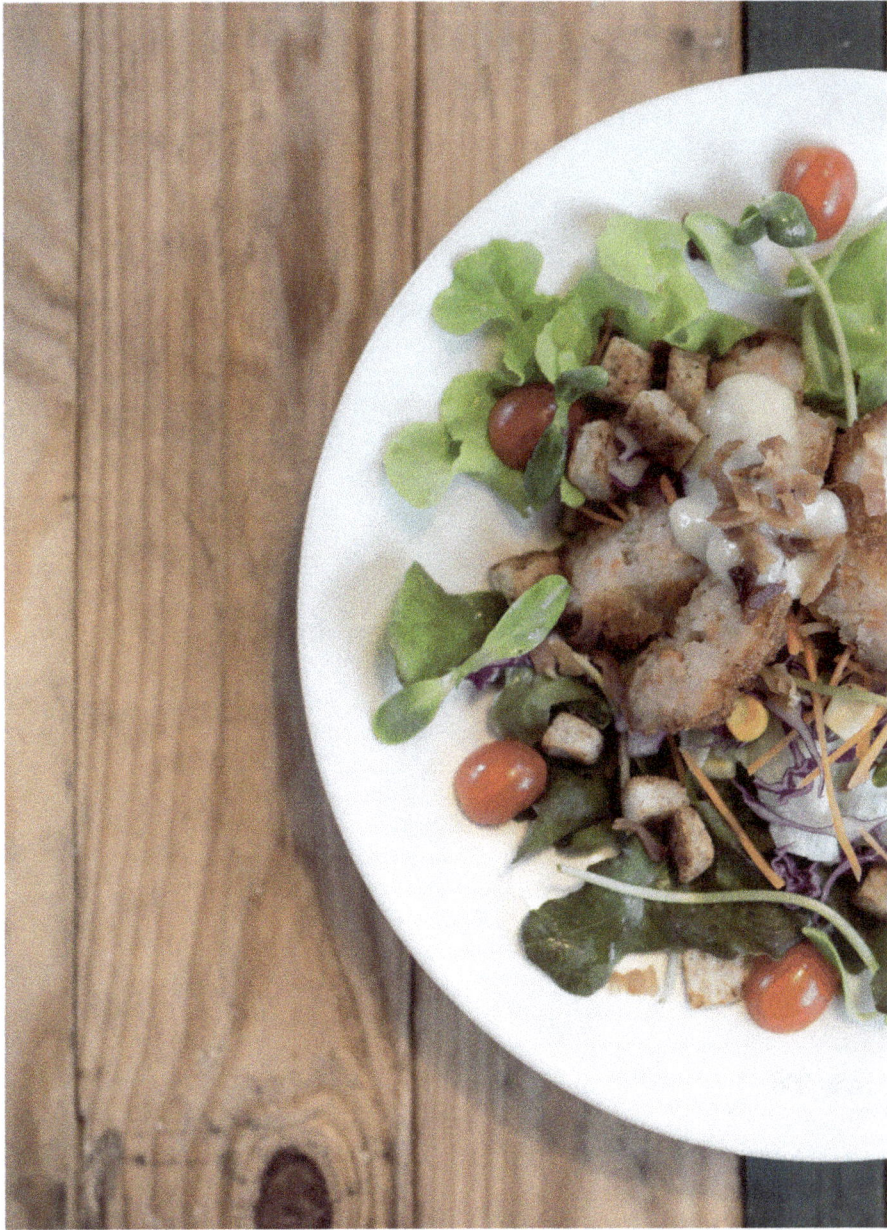

Passionate Quinoa and Black Bean Salad

Serving: 6

Prep Time: 5 minutes

Cook Time: 15 minutes

Ingredients:

1 cup uncooked quinoa

1 can 15 ounce black beans, drained and rinsed 1/3 cup cilantro, chopped

1 tablespoon olive oil

1 clove garlic, minced

Juice from 1 lime

Salt and pepper as needed

How To:

1.	Cook quinoa according to the package instructions.

2.	Transfer quinoa to a medium bowl and let it cool for 10 minutes.

3.   Add remaining ingredients and toss well.

4.   Serve and enjoy!

Nutrition (Per Serving)

Calories: 188

Fat: 4g

Carbohydrates: 29g

Protein: 8g

Zucchini Noodle Salad

Serving: 3

Prep Time: 15 minutes

Cook Time: nil

Ingredients:

2 large zucchini, spiralized/peeled into thin strips

1 small tomato, diced

¼ red onion, sliced thinly

1 large avocado, diced

½ cup olive oil

¼ cup balsamic vinegar

1 garlic clove, minced

2 teaspoons Dijon mustard

Salt and pepper to taste

¼ cup blue cheese, crumbles

How To:

1.   Take a large bowl and add zucchini noodles, onion, tomato, avocado.

2.   Take a small bowl and whisk in olive oil, vinegar, mustard, garlic, salt and pepper.

3.   Drizzle over salad and toss.

4.   Divide into serving bowls and top with blue cheese crumbles.

5.   Enjoy!

Nutrition (Per Serving)

Calories: 770

Fat: 74

Carbohydrates: 12g

Protein: 8g

Onion and Orange Healthy Salad

Serving: 3

Prep Time: 10 minutes

Cook Time: nil

Ingredients:

6 large oranges

3 tablespoons red wine vinegar

6 tablespoons olive oil

1 teaspoon dried oregano

1 red onion, thinly sliced

1 cup olive oil

¼ cup fresh chives, chopped Ground black pepper

How To:

1.   Peel the oranges and cut each of them in 4-5 crosswise slices.

2.   Transfer the oranges to a shallow dish.

3.   Drizzle vinegar, olive oil and sprinkle oregano.

4.   Toss.

5.   Chill for 30 minutes.

6.   Arrange sliced onion and black olives on top.

7.   Decorate with additional sprinkle of chives and fresh grind of pepper.

8.   Serve and enjoy!

Nutrition (Per Serving)

Calories: 120

Fat: 6g

Carbohydrates: 20g

Protein: 2g

Stir Fried Almond and Spinach

Serving: 2

Prep Time: 10 minutes

Cook Time: 15 minutes

Ingredients:

34 pounds spinach

3 tablespoons almonds

Salt to taste

1 tablespoon coconut oil

How To:

1.   Add oil to a large pot and place on high heat.

2.   Add spinach and let it cook, stirring frequently.

3.   Once the spinach is cooked and tender, season with salt and stir.

4.   Add almonds and enjoy!

Nutrition (Per Serving)

Calories: 150

Fat: 12g

Carbohydrates: 10g

Protein: 8g

Cilantro and Avocado Platter

Serving: 6

Prep Time: 10 minutes

Cook Time: nil

Ingredients:

2 avocados, peeled, pitted and diced

1 sweet onion, chopped

1 green bell pepper, chopped

1 large ripe tomato, chopped

¼ cup fresh cilantro, chopped

½ lime, juiced

Salt and pepper as needed

How To:

1.   Take a medium sized owl and add onion, bell pepper, tomato, avocados, lime and cilantro.

2.   Mix well and give it a toss.

3.   Season with salt and pepper according to your taste.

4. Serve and enjoy!

Nutrition (Per Serving)

Calories: 126

Fat: 10g

Carbohydrates: 10g

Protein: 2g

Chicken Breast Salad

Serving: 4

Prep Time: 25 minutes

Cook Time: 30-55 minutes

Ingredients:

3 ½ ounces chicken breast

2 tablespoons spinach

1 ¾ ounces lettuces

1 bell pepper

2 tablespoons olive oil

Lemon juice to taste

How To:

1.   Boil chicken breast without adding salt, cut the meat into small strips.

2.   Put the spinach in boiling water for a few minutes, cut into small strips.

3.   Cut pepper in strips as well.

4.   Add everything to a bowl and mix with juice and oil.

5.   Serve!

Nutrition (Per Serving)

Calories: 100

Fat: 11g

Carbohydrates: 3g

Protein: 6g

Broccoli Salad

Serving: 1

Prep Time: 5 minutes

Cook Time: 10 minutes

Ingredients:

broccoli florets

2 red onions, sliced

1-ounce bacon, chopped into small pieces

1 cup coconut cream

1 teaspoon sesame seeds Salt

How To:

1.   Cook bacon in hot oil until crispy.

2.   Cook onions in fat left from the bacon.

3.   Take a pan of boiling water and add broccoli florets, boil for a few minutes.

4.   Take a salad bowl and add bacon pieces, onions, broccoli florets, coconut cream and salt.

5.   Toss well and top with sesame seeds.

6. Enjoy!

Nutrition (Per Serving)

Calories: 280

Fat: 26g

Carbohydrates: 8g

Protein: 10g

Hearty Quinoa and Fruit Salad

Serving: 5

Prep Time: 5 minutes

Cook Time: 10 minutes

Ingredients:

3 ½ ounces Quinoa

3 peaches, diced

1 ½ ounces toasted hazelnuts, chopped

Handful of mint, chopped

Handful of parsley, chopped

2 tablespoons olive oil

Zest of 1 lemon

Juice of 1 lemon

How To:

1.   Take medium sized saucepan and add quinoa.

2.   Add 1 ¼ cups of water and bring it to a boil over medium-high heat.

3.   Reduce the heat to low and simmer for 20 minutes.

4.   Drain any excess liquid.

5.   Add fruits, herbs, hazelnuts to the quinoa.

6.   Allow it to cool and season.

7.   Take a bowl and add olive oil, lemon zest and lemon juice.

8.   Pour the mixture over the salad and give it a mix.

9.   Enjoy!

Nutrition (Per Serving)

Calories: 148

Fat: 8g

Carbohydrates: 16g

Protein: 5g

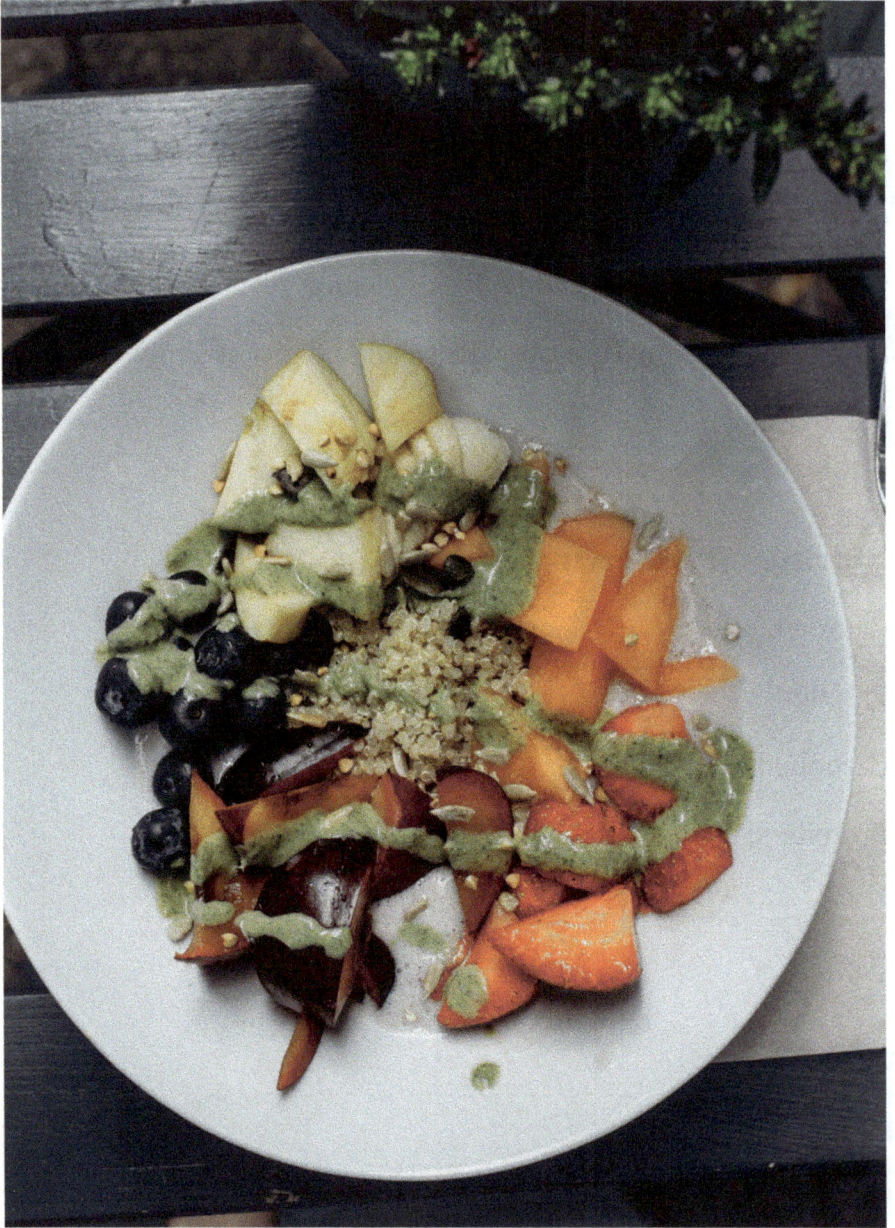

Amazing Quinoa and Black Bean Salad

Serving: 4

Prep Time: 5 minutes

Cook Time: 2-3 minutes

Ingredients:

1 cup uncooked quinoa

1 can 15-ounce black beans, drained and rinsed 1/3 cup cilantro, chopped

1 tablespoon olive oil

1 clove garlic, minced

Juice from 1 lime

Salt and pepper as needed

How To:

1.   Cook quinoa according to package instructions.

2.   Transfer quinoa to a medium bowl and allow it to cool for 10 minutes.

3.   Add the rest of the ingredients and toss.

4. Serve and enjoy!

5. Enjoy!

Nutrition (Per Serving)

Calories: 188

Fat: 4g

Carbohydrates: 29g

Protein: 8g

Authentic Mediterranean Pearl and Couscous

Serving: 4

Prep Time: 15 minutes

Cook Time: 10 minutes

Ingredients:

For the Vinaigrette

1 large lemon, juiced

1/3 cup extra virgin olive oil

1 teaspoon dill weed

1 teaspoon garlic powder

Salt and pepper as needed

For Israeli Couscous

2 cups Pearl Couscous

Extra virgin olive oil

2 cups grape tomatoes, halved

Water as needed

1/3 cup red onions, chopped

½ English Cucumber, chopped

15 ounces chickpeas

14 ounce (can) fresh artichoke hearts, chopped ½ cup kalamata olives, pitted

15-20 pieces fresh basil leaves, torn and chopped

3 ounces fresh baby mozzarella cheese

How To:

1.   Start by preparing the vinaigrette. Take a bowl and add the ingredients listed under vinaigrette.

2.   Mix them well and keep it on the side.

3.   Take a medium sized heavy pot and place it over medium heat.

4.   Add 2 tablespoons of olive oil and allow it to heat up.

5.   Add couscous and keep cooking until golden brown.

6.   Add 3 cups of boiling water and cook the couscous according to package instructions.

7.   Once done, drain in a colander and keep on the side.

8.   Take another large sized mixing bowl and add the rest of the ingredients, except cheese and basil.

9.   Add the cooked couscous and basil to the mix and mix everything well.

10. Give the vinaigrette a nice stir and whisk it into the couscous salad.

11. Mix well.

12. Adjust the seasoning as required.

13. Add mozzarella cheese.

14. Garnish with some basil.

15. Enjoy!

Nutrition (Per Serving)

Calories: 393

Fat: 13g

Carbohydrates: 57g

Protein: 13g

Mesmerizing Fruit Bowl

Serving: 1

Prep Time: 30 minutes

Cook Time: nil

Ingredients:

2 fresh ripe mangoes

2 cups pineapple chunks

Fresh pineapple tips

1 banana, sliced

1-2 cups fresh papaya, cubed

1 kiwi fruit, cubed

2 cups seedless grapes, halved

¼ cup coconut milk

2 tablespoons lime juice

3-4 tablespoons sugar

Strawberries, cranberries or raspberries as topping

How To:

1.   Slice the fruits above, except the contrasting red ones such as dried cranberries, raspberries and strawberries.

2.   Add them to your mixing bowl and drizzle a bit of lime juice on top.

3.   Stir well and sprinkle a bit of sugar on top, give it a nice stir.

4.   Allow it to chill for 30 minutes and serve the salad with a bit of coconut milk.

5.   Season the sweetness accordingly and top it with some cranberries, raspberries and strawberries.

6.   Enjoy!

Nutrition (Per Serving)

Calories: 209

Fat: 0g

Carbohydrates: 43g

Protein: 2g

Tangy Strawberry Salad

Serving: 4

Prep Time: 15 minutes

Cook Time: nil

Ingredients:

4 slices bacon, cooked and crumbled

10 large strawberries, stem removed and sliced

4 cups baby spinach

1 avocado, chopped

For Dressing

Zest of 1 lemon

¼ red onion, minced

¼ cup red wine vinegar

1 tablespoon Dijon mustard

1 lemon, juiced

1 teaspoon poppy seed

½ cup extra light olive oil

How To:

1.   Add all the dressing ingredients to a blender and blend until you have a smooth mixture (except poppy seeds).

2.   Stir in poppy seeds after blending.

3.   Take a large bowl and toss strawberries, bacon, spinach and avocado.

4.   Mix well and drizzle the dressing on top.

5.   Serve and enjoy!

Nutrition (Per Serving)

Calories: 96

Fat: 1g

Carbohydrates: 22g

Protein: 3g

Peachful Applesauce Salad

Serving: 6

Prep Time: 15 minutes

Cook Time: nil

Ingredients:

1 cup diet lemon lime-soda

1 pack sugar-free fruit mixed peach gelatin

1 cup unsweetened applesauce

2 cups coconut whip cream

1/8 teaspoon ground nutmeg

1/8 teaspoon vanilla extract

1 fresh peach, peeled and chopped

How To:

1.   Take a saucepan and bring the soda to a boil over medium heat.

2.   Remove heat.

3.   Stir in sugar-free peach gelatin until dissolved.

4. Add applesauce and stir.

5. Let it chill until partially set.

6. Fold in whipped topping and vanilla extract.

7. Fold in the peach and wait until firm.

8. Serve and enjoy!

Nutrition (Per Serving)

Calories: 354

Fat: 17g

Carbohydrates: 37g

Protein: 15g

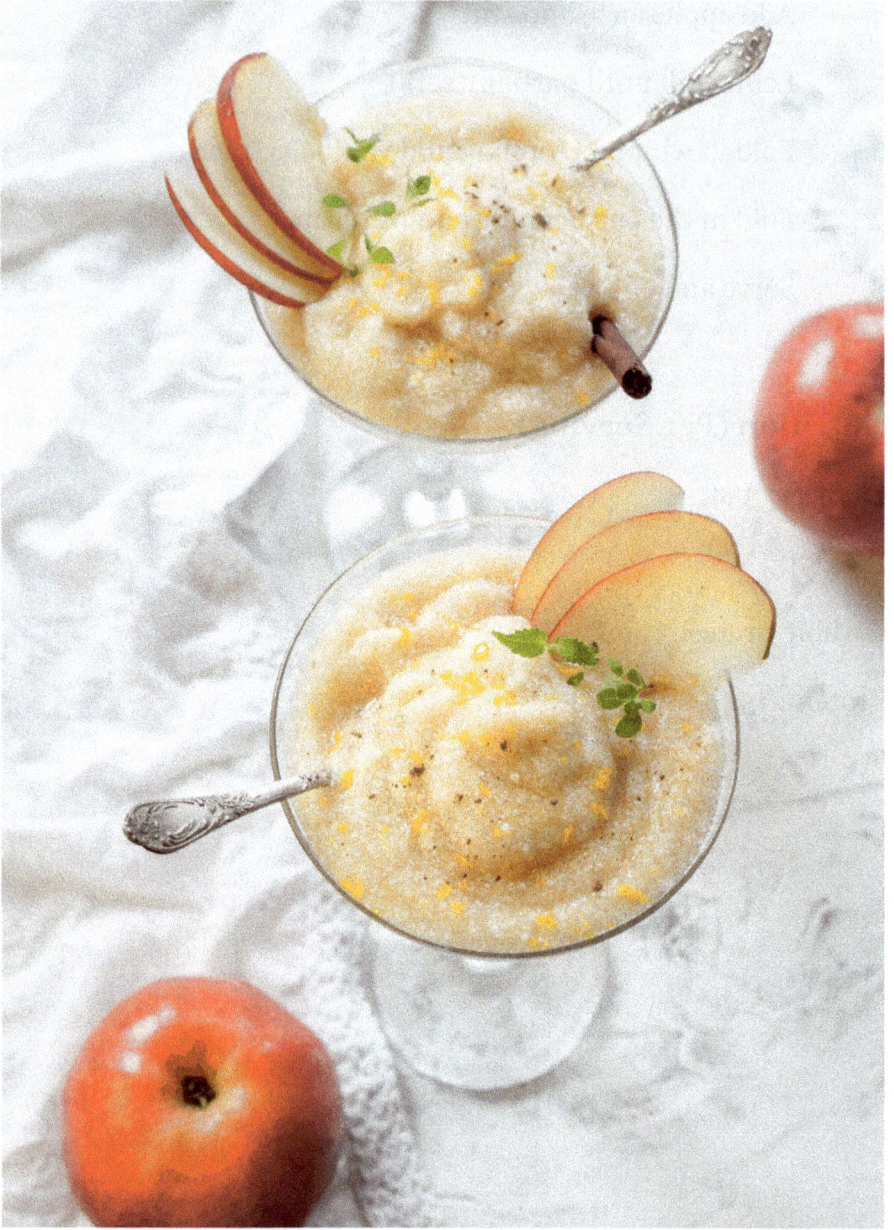

The Citrus Lover's Salad

Serving: 16

Prep Time: 10 minutes

Cook Time: nil

Ingredients:

1 medium zucchini, julienned

½ cup olive oil

1 medium red onion, sliced

1 cup fresh broccoli, cut into florets

1 cup fresh cauliflower florets

1/8 teaspoon pepper

1 medium cucumber, halved and sliced ¼ cup white wine vinegar

1 teaspoon dried oregano

1 medium carrot, julienned

½ teaspoon ground mustard

¼ teaspoon garlic powder

1/8 teaspoon celery salt

How To:

1. Add olives and veggies to a small bowl.

2. Take another bowl and whisk in vinegar, seasoning, oil.

3. Pour the mixture over veggies and toss.

4. Let sit for 3 hours.

5. Serve and enjoy!

Nutrition (Per Serving)

Calories: 72

Fat: 7g

Carbohydrates: 2g

Protein: 2g

Wicked Vanilla Fruit Salad

Serving: 5

Prep Time: 10 minutes

Cook Time: nil

Ingredients:

8 cans mandarin orange, drained

4 packs instant vanilla pudding mix

6 cans pineapple chunks

10 medium red apples, chopped

How To:

1.   Drain pineapples, making sure to reserve the liquid.

2.   Keep them on the side.

3.   Add cold water to the juice to make 6 cups liquid in total.

4.   Whisk the juice mix and pudding mix into a large bowl for about 2 minutes.

5.   Let it stand for 2 minutes until soft-set.

6.   Stir in apples, oranges and reserved pineapple.

7. Chill in fridge and serve.

8. Enjoy!

Nutrition (Per Serving)

Calories: 33

Fat: 0g

Carbohydrates: 8g

Protein: 0g

Green Papaya Salad

Serving: 6

Prep Time: 10 minutes

Cook Time: nil

Ingredients:

10 small shrimps, dried

2 small red Thai Chilies

1 garlic clove, peeled

¼ cup tamarind juice

1 tablespoon palm sugar

1 tablespoon Thai fish sauce, low sodium

1 lime, cut into 1-inch pieces

4 cherry tomatoes, halved

3 long beans, trimmed into 1-inch pieces

1 carrot, coarsely shredded

½ English cucumber, coarsely chopped and seeded 1/6 small green cabbage, cored and thinly sliced

1-pound unripe green papaya, quartered, seeded and shredded using a mandolin

3 tablespoons unsalted roasted peanuts

How To:

1.   Take a mortar and pestle and crush your shrimp alongside garlic, chilies.

2.   Add tamarind juice, fish sauce and palm sugar.

3.   Squeeze the juice from the lime pieces and pour 3 quarts over the mortar.

4.   Grind the mixture in the mortar to make a dressing, keep the dressing on the side.

5.   Take a bowl, add the remaining ingredients (excluding the peanut), making sure to add the papaya last.

6.   Use a spoon and stir in the dressing.

7.   Mix the vegetables and fruit and coat them well.

8.   Transfer to your serving dish.

9.   Garnish with some peanuts and lime pieces.

10.   Enjoy!

Nutrition (Per Serving)

Calories: 316

Fat: 13g

Carbohydrates: 5g

Protein: 11g

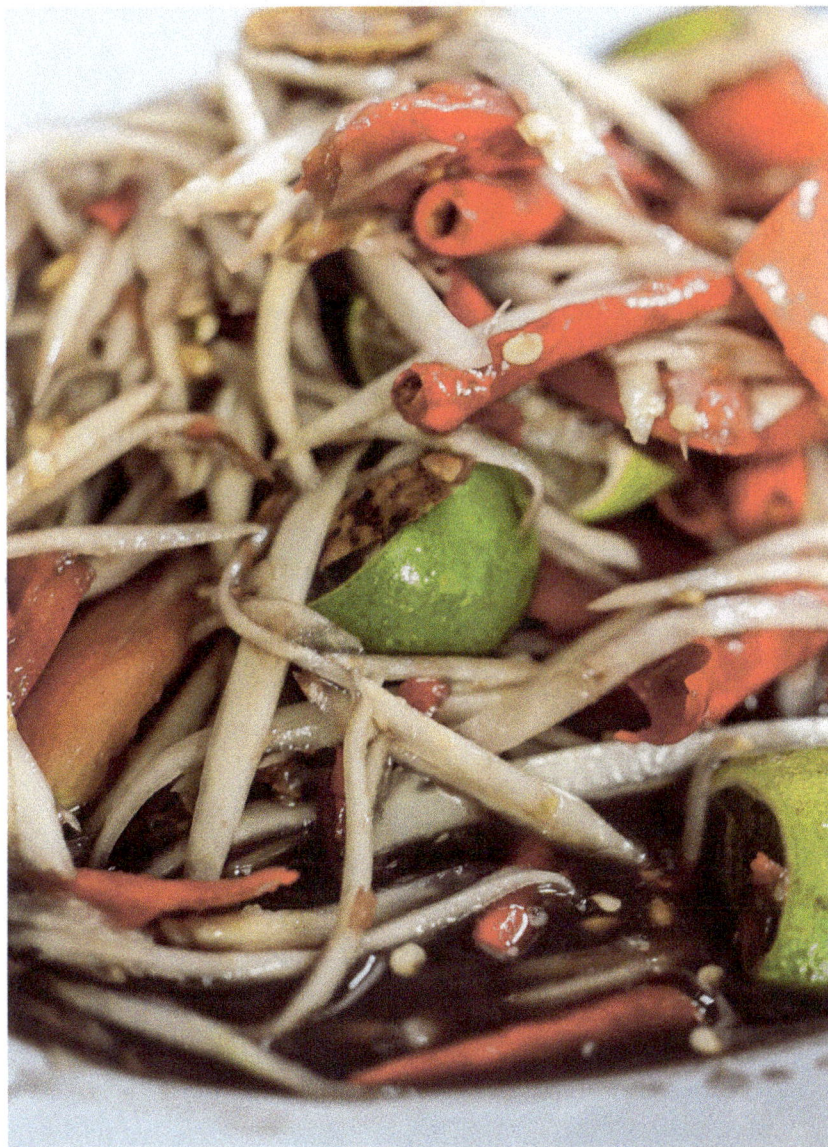

Pineapple, Papaya and Mango Delight

Serving: 2

Prep Time: 20 minutes

Cook Time: nil

Ingredients:

1-pound fresh pineapple, peeled and cut into chunks mango, peeled, pitted and cubed papayas, peeled, seeded and cubed

tablespoons fresh lime juice

¼ cup fresh mint leaves, chopped

How To:

1. Take a large bowl and add the listed ingredients.

2.   Toss well to coat.

3.   Put in fridge and chill. Serve and enjoy!

Nutrition (Per Serving)

Calories: 292

Fat: 11g

Carbohydrates: 42g

Protein: 8g

Cashew and Green Apple Salad

Serving: 2

Prep Time: 15 minutes

Cook Time: nil

Ingredients:

½ large apple, cored and sliced

2 cups mixed fresh greens

1 tablespoon unsalted cashews

1 tablespoon apple cider vinegar

How To:

1.   Take a serving bowl and add apple, cashews and greens.

2.   Drizzle apple cider vinegar on top.

3.   Serve immediately!

Nutrition (Per Serving)

Calories: 118

Fat: 4g

Carbohydrates: 19g

Protein: 3g

Watermelon and Tomato Mix

Serving: 2

Prep Time: 20 minutes

Cook Time: nil

Ingredients:

1 large red tomato, cubed

1 large yellow tomato, cubed

2 cups fresh watermelon, peeled, seeded and cubed

Dressing

¼ cup olive oil

¼ cup rice wine vinegar

2 teaspoons honey

2 tablespoons chili garlic sauce

1 tablespoon fresh lemon basil, chopped Salt and pepper as needed

How To:

1.   Take a large bowl and add all the salad ingredients.

2.   Take another bowl and add the dressing ingredients.

3.   Beat well until combined.

4.   Pour dressing over salad and toss.

5.   Serve and enjoy!

Nutrition (Per Serving)

Calories: 87

Fat: 7g

Carbohydrates: 7g

Protein: 0.6g

Low Sodium Sheet Pan Chicken Fajitas

Ingredients

Two lbs chicken breast tenderloin each sliced in half lengthwise

One green pepper sliced

One red bell pepper sliced

One Vidalia onion sliced

Olive oil spray

One tablespoon olive oil Seasoning:

One teaspoon chili powder

1/2 teaspoon smoked paprika

1/2 teaspoon garlic powder 1/2 teaspoon onion powder 1/2 teaspoon dried oregano

1/2 teaspoon dried cilantro

1/2 teaspoon cumin

1/4 teaspoon cayenne pepper

Instructions

1.   Preheat oven to 350 degrees F.

2.   Apply a coat on a sheet pan with vegetable oil spray.

3.   Spread pepper and onion slices onto a prepared sheet pan.

4.   Place chicken slices on top of vegetables.

5.   Combine seasoning ingredients and stir to mix.

6.   Drizzle seasoning mixture over chicken, peppers, and onion.

7.   Sprinkle 1 tbsp of vegetable oil over chicken, peppers, and onion.

8.   Gently toss ingredients to distribute seasoning and oil evenly. (make sure chicken strips aren't overlapping)

9.   Bake for 20 min or until chicken reaches 165 deg F.

10.   Serve in warm low sodium tortillas.

11.   Top together with your favorite toppings! i really like cheddar and soured cream.

Nutrition Facts

Calories 168Calories from Fat 36 Fat 4g6% Sodium 140mg6% Potassium 531mg15% Carbohydrates 5g2% Fiber 1g4% Sugar 3g3% Protein 24g48%

Vitamin C 34.3mg42% Calcium 17mg2% Iron 0.8mg4%

Pineapple Protein Smoothie Ingredients

3/4 cup milk

3/4 cup pineapple chunks

1/2 cup ice

3/4 cup canned chickpeas (rinsed and drained)

2 tbsp almond butter

Two pitted dates

2 tsp ground turmeric

Directions

Blend all ingredients until smooth.

Nutrients Calories: 461

Spinach Sunshine Smoothie Bowl

Ingredients

One packed cup baby spinach

One banana

1 cup of orange juice

1/2 avocado

1/2 cup ice cubes

Blueberries (optional)

Diced pineapple (optional)

Ground flaxseeds (optional)

Directions

Process the spinach, banana, fruit juice, avocado, and ice during a blender until very smooth.

Serve topped with blueberries, diced pineapple, and ground flaxseeds.

Almond Butter Berry Smoothie

Ingredients

1/4 cup 1% low-fat milk

1/2 medium ripe banana

1 tbsp creamy almond butter

1 cup fresh or frozen raspberries

1/2 cup crushed ice

Directions

Blend all ingredients until smooth and enjoy!

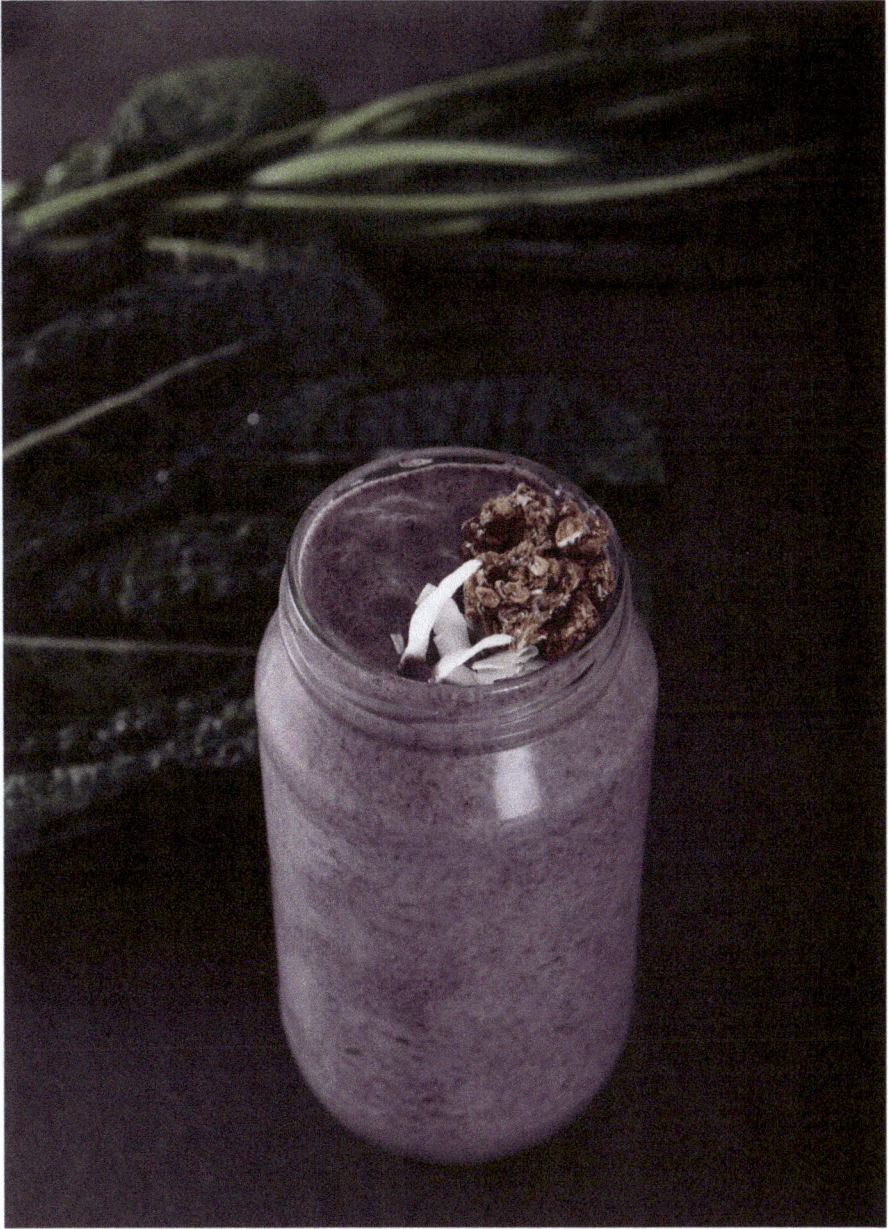

Pomegranate and Peaches Avocado Toast

Ingredients

one slice whole-grain bread

1/2 avocado

1 tbsp ricotta

Pomegranate seeds, a small amount like one handful Drizzle honey

Directions

1.   Toast the entire grain bread within the oven or toaster.

2.   Spread avocado onto the toast, as smooth or coarse as you favor.

3.   Spread a dollop of ricotta across the avocado.

4.   Drizzle a piece of honey over the avocado mixture.

5.   Sprinkle pomegranate seeds on top and luxuriate in.

Breakfast in a Jar

Ingredients

1/4 cup of oatmeal

3/4 cup of kefir

1 tbsp of chia seeds

2 tbsp of raisins

1 tbsp of unsweetened coconut flakes

Instructions

Make Layers of elements during a 16-ounce Mason jar , close the lid and refrigerate overnight.

When it's able to eat, remove the jar from the fridge and provides it a fast stir.

Avocado Egg Cups

Ingredients

Two avocados, ripe

1/4 tsp coarse salt

1/4 tsp pepper

1/2 tsp olive oil

Four medium eggs

1 tbsp grated cheese, such as Parmesan, cheddar, or Swiss
Assorted toppings: herbs, scallions, salsa, diced tomato, crumbled bacon, Sriracha, paprika, crumbled feta

Directions

1.   Heat oven to 375°F. Halve avocados lengthwise and pit. Cut a thin slice from bottom of every avocado half so that it sits level. Where Hell was, scoop out only enough of the flesh (about ½ tbsp) to form room for an egg.

2.   Place avocados on a foil-lined rimmed baking sheet. Season each with salt and pepper, and rub with vegetable oil.

3.   Crack an egg into each cavity (some of the albumen will run over the side, but don't be concerned about it). Sprinkle with cheese, if using. Cover loosely with foil.

4.   Bake almost 20 to 25 min, or until eggs are set to your liking. Sprinkle with toppings.

Coconut Oil Fat Bombs

Ingredients

Coconut oil-1 1/2 tbsp-20.8 grams

Cocoa-Dry powder, unsweetened-3/4 tbsp-4.1 grams

Honey-5/16 tsp-2 grams

Salt-Table-1/8 tsp-0.57 grams

Directions

1.   Mix all the ingredients during a processor until the mixture is smooth and creamy.

2.   Pour into small-sized cube trays or silicone moulds and freeze.

3.   Once frozen, pop the copra oil fat bombs out of the pictures and store them during a freezer zip-top bag or jar. Enjoy!

Nutrition

Calories 194 Carbs 4g Fat 21g Protein 1g Fiber 2g Net carbs 3g Sodium 222mg Cholesterol 0mg

Apricot Jam and Almond Butter Sandwich

Ingredients

Multi-grain bread-Two slices regular-52 grams Jams and preserves-1 tbsp-20 grams

Almond butter-Nuts, every day, without salt, added-1 tbsp-16 grams

Directions

1.   Toast the bread optionally.

2.   Spread almond butter on one side and jam on the other side.

Nutrition

Calories 292 Carbs 39g Fat 11g Protein 10g Fiber 6g Net carbs 34g Sodium 206mg Cholesterol 0mg

Peanut Butter and Honey Toast

Ingredients

Multi-grain bread-Two slices regular-52 grams

Peanut butter-Smooth style, without salt-3 tbsp-48 grams

Honey-2 tbsp-42 grams

Directions

1.   Toast the bread, and it is optionally.

2.   Spread peanut butter on the bread and sprinkle with honey. Enjoy!

Nutrition

Calories 553 Carbs 68g Fat 27g Protein 18g Fiber 6g Net carbs 62g Sodium 208mg Cholesterol 0mg

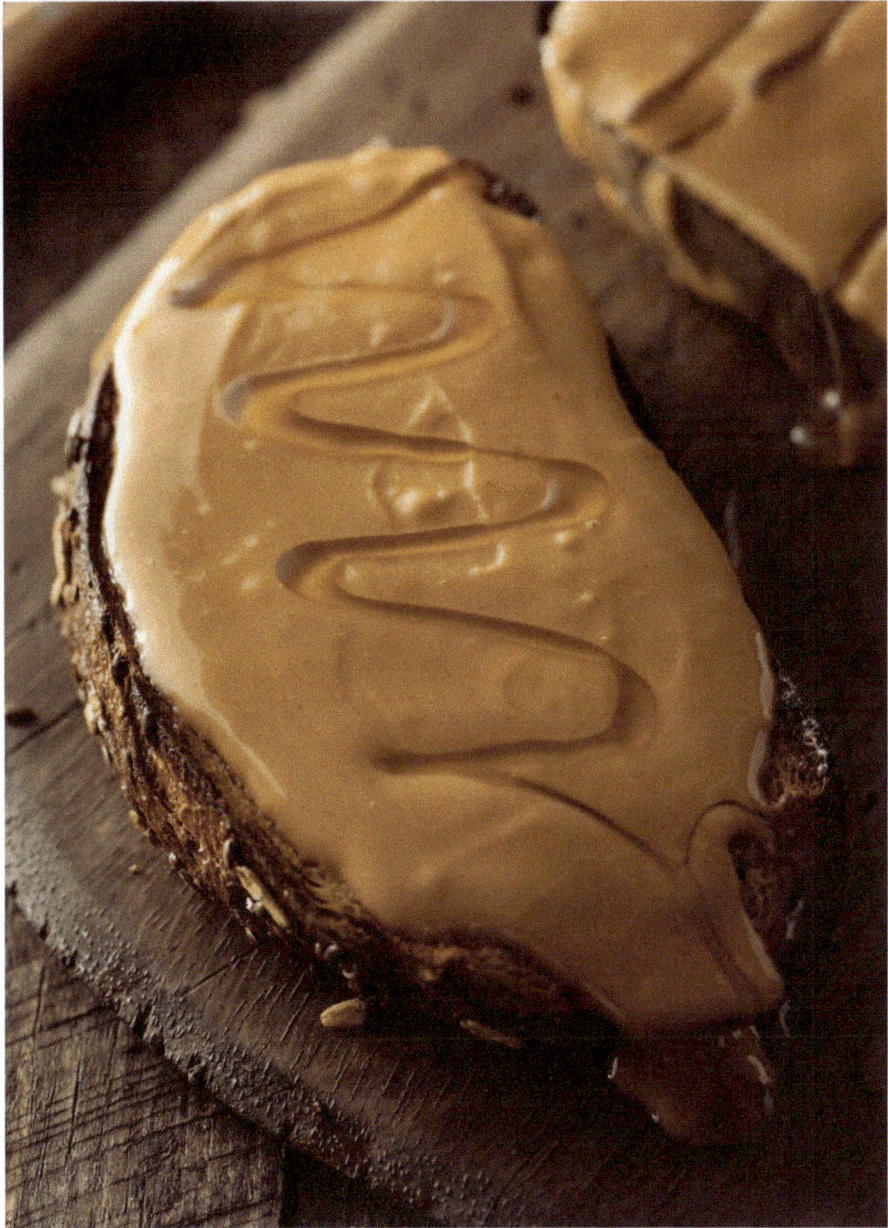

Cucumber & Hummus

Ingredients

Hummus-Commercial-1/4 cup-61.5 grams Cucumber-With peel, raw-1 cup slices-104 grams

Directions

Cut the cucumber into round slices and eat with hummus.

Nutrition

Calories 118

Carbs13g

Fat6g

Protein6g

Fiber4g

Net carbs8g

Carrot and Hummus Snack

Ingredients

Hummus-Commercial-2 tbsp-30 grams Baby carrots-Baby, raw-1 cup-246 grams

Directions

Dip carrots into hummus and enjoy!

Nutrition

Calories136Carbs25gFat3gProtein4gFiber9gNet

carbs16gSodium306mgCholesterol0mg

Yogurt with Walnuts & Honey

Ingredients

Walnuts-Nuts, black, dried-1/4 cup, chopped-31.3 grams

Non-fat greek yoghurt-Nonfat, plain-480cup-480 grams

Honey-2 tsp-14.1 gram

Directions

1.   Rough-chop walnuts and mix into yogurt.

2.   Top with honey and enjoy!

Nutrition

Calories520Carbs32gFat20gProtein56gFiber2gNet

carbs30gSodium174mgCholesterol24mg

Chicken Veggie Packets

Ingredients

Four boneless and skinless chicken breast halves (4 ounces each) 1/2 pound sliced fresh mushrooms 1-1/2 cups fresh baby carrots

1 cup pearl onions

1/2 cup julienned sweet red pepper

1/4 teaspoon pepper

Three teaspoons minced fresh thyme

1/2 teaspoon salt, optional

Lemon wedges, optional

Directions

1.   Flatten bird breasts to 1/2-in. Thickness; vicinity every on a touch of industrial quality foil (about 12 in. Square). Layer the mushrooms, carrots, onions and pink pepper over bird; sprinkle with pepper, thyme and salt if desired.

2.   Fold foil around hen and greens and seal tightly. Place on a baking sheet. Bake at 375° for a half-hour or until chook juices run clear. If desired, serve with lemon wedges.

Nutrition Facts

175 calories, 3g fat (1g saturated fat), 63mg cholesterol, 100mg sodium, 11g carbohydrate (6g sugars, 2g fibre), 25g protein.

Sweet Onion & Sausage Spaghetti

Ingredients

6 ounces uncooked whole-wheat spaghetti

3/4pound Italian turkey sausage links, casings removed Two teaspoons olive oil

One sweet onion, thinly sliced

1-pint cherry tomatoes halved

One and a half cup of fresh basil leaves (sliced)

1/2 cup half-and-half cream

Shaved Parmesan cheese, optional

Directions

1.   Cook spaghetti consistent with directions given. At an equivalent time, during a large nonstick skillet over medium heat, cook sausage in oil for five minutes. Add onion; bake 8-10 minutes longer or until meat is not any longer pink and onion is tender.

2.   Stir in tomatoes and basil; heat through. Add cream; bring back a boil. Drain spaghetti; toss with sausage mixture. Garnish with cheese if desired.

Nutrition Facts

334 calories, 12g fat (4g saturated fat), 46mg cholesterol, 378mg sodium, 41g carbohydrate (8g sugars, 6g fibre), 17g protein.

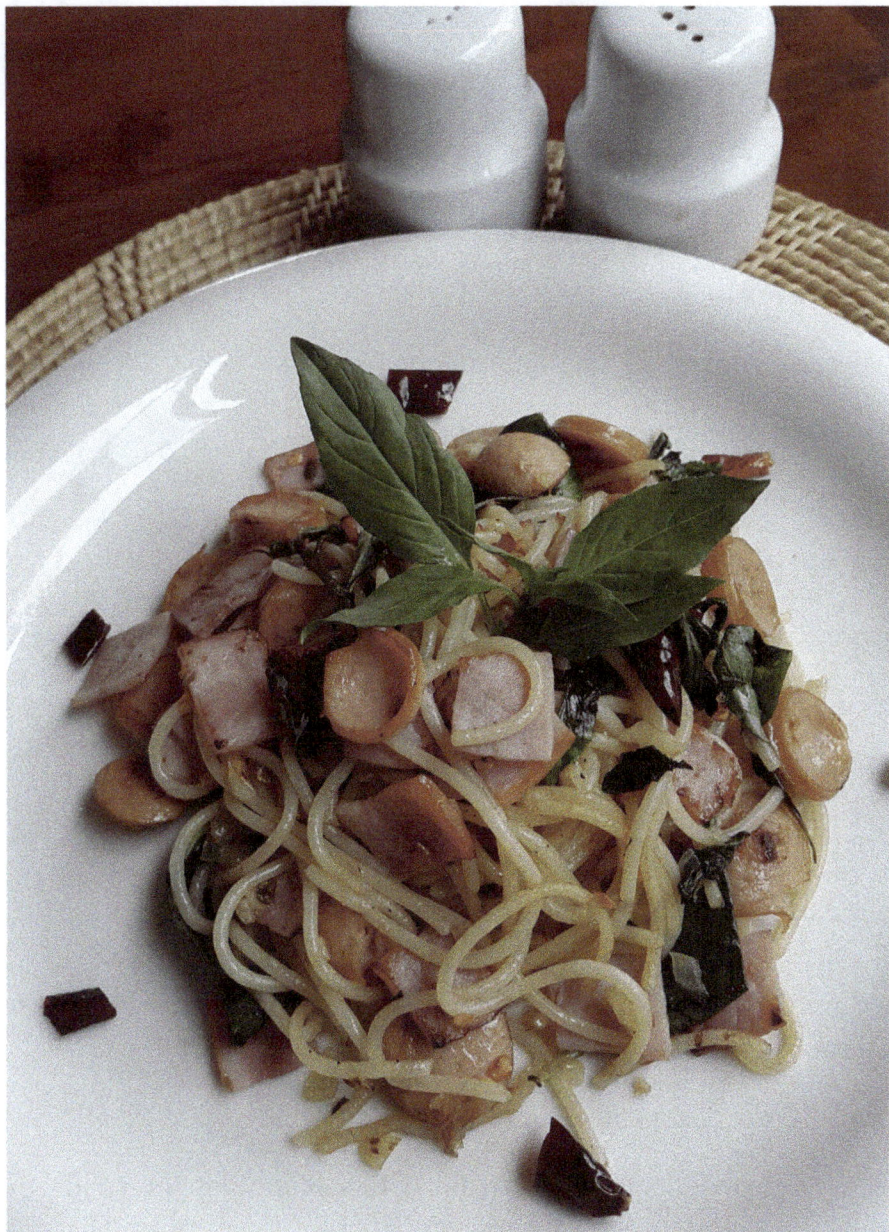

Beef and Blue Cheese Penne with Pesto

Ingredients

2 cups uncooked whole wheat penne pasta

Two beef tenderloin steaks (6 ounces each)

1/4 teaspoon salt

1/4 teaspoon pepper

5 ounces of fresh baby spinach (about 6 cups), coarsely chopped

2 cups grape tomatoes, halved

1/3 cup prepared pesto

1/4 cup chopped walnuts

1/4 cup crumbled Gorgonzola cheese

Directions

1. Cook pasta consistent with package directions.

2. Meanwhile, sprinkle steaks with salt and pepper. Grill steaks, covered, over medium heat. Heat for 5-7 mins on all sides or until meat reaches desired doneness.

3.   Drain pasta; transfer to an outsized bowl. Add spinach, tomatoes, pesto and walnuts; toss to coat. Cut steak into thin slices. Serve pasta mixture with beef; sprinkle with cheese.

Nutrition Facts

532 calories, 22g fat (6g saturated fat), 50mg cholesterol, 434mg sodium, 49g carbohydrate (3g sugars, 9g fibre), 35g protein.

Asparagus Turkey Stir-Fry

Ingredients

Two teaspoons cornstarch

1/4 cup chicken broth

One tablespoon lemon juice

One teaspoon soy sauce

1 pound of turkey breast tenderloins, cut into 1/2-inch strips
One garlic clove, minced

Two tablespoons canola oil, divided

1 pound of asparagus, cut into 1-1/2-inch pieces One jar (2 ounces) sliced pimientos, drained

Instructions

1.   In a little bowl, mix the cornstarch, broth, juice and soy until smooth; put aside. during a large skillet or wok, stir-fry turkey and garlic in 1 tablespoon oil until meat is not any longer pink; remove and keep warm.

2.   Stir-fry asparagus in remaining oil until crisp-tender. Add pimientos. Stir the mixture and increase the pan; cook and stir for 1 minute or until thickened. Return turkey to the pan; heat through.

Nutrition Facts

205 calories, 9g fat (1g saturated fat), 56mg cholesterol, 204mg sodium, 5g carbohydrate (1g sugars, 1g fiber), 28g protein.

Chicken with Celery Root Puree

Ingredients

Four boneless skinless chicken breast halves (6 ounces each)

1/2 teaspoon pepper

1/4 teaspoon salt

Three teaspoons canola oil, divided

One large celery root, peeled and chopped (about 3 cups)

2 cups diced peeled butternut squash

One small onion, chopped

Two garlic cloves, minced

2/3 cup unsweetened apple juice

Instructions

1.   Sprinkle chicken with pepper and salt. Take an outsized skillet and coat with cooking spray, heat two teaspoons oil over medium heat. Brown chicken on each side. Remove chicken from pan.

2.   Heat the remaining oil over medium-high within the same pan. Add celery root, squash and onion; cook and stir until squash is crisp-tender. Add garlic; cook 1 minute longer.

3.   Return chicken to pan; add fruit juice. bring back a boil. Reduce heat; simmer, covered, 12-15 minutes or until a thermometer inserted in chicken reads 165°.

4.   Remove chicken; keep warm. Cool vegetable mixture slightly. Process during a kitchen appliance until smooth. Return to pan and warmth through. Serve with chicken.

Nutrition Facts

328 calories, 8g fat (1g saturated fat), 94mg cholesterol, 348mg sodium, 28g carbohydrate (10g sugars, 5g fibre), 37g protein.

Wholesome Potato and Tuna Salad

Serving: 4

Prep Time: 10 minutes

Cook Time: nil

Ingredients:

1 pound baby potatoes, scrubbed, boiled

1 cup tuna chunks, drained

1 cup cherry tomatoes, halved

1 cup medium onion, thinly sliced

8 pitted black olives

2 medium hard-boiled eggs, sliced

1 head Romaine lettuce

¼ cup olive oil

2 tablespoons lemon juice

1 tablespoon Dijon mustard

1 teaspoon dill weed, chopped Pepper as needed

How To:

1.   Take a small glass bowl and mix in your olive oil, lemon juice, Dijon mustard and dill.

2.   Season the mix with pepper and salt.

3.   Add in the tuna, baby potatoes, cherry tomatoes, red onion, green beans, black olives and toss everything nicely.

4.   Arrange your lettuce leaves on a beautiful serving dish to make the base of your salad.

5.   Top them with your salad mixture and place the egg slices.

6.   Drizzle with the previously prepared Salad Dressing.

7.   Serve hot

Nutrition (Per Serving)

Calories: 406

Fat: 22g

Carbohydrates: 28g

Protein: 26g

Baby Spinach Salad

Serving: 2

Prep Time: 10 minutes

Cook Time: nil

Ingredients:

1 bag baby spinach, washed and dried

1 red bell pepper, cut in slices

1 cup cherry tomatoes, cut in halves

1 small red onion, finely chopped

1 cup black olives, pitted

For dressing:

1 teaspoon dried oregano

1 large garlic clove

3 tablespoons red wine vinegar

4 tablespoons olive oil

Sunflower seeds and pepper to taste

How To:

1.   Prepare the dressing by blending in garlic, olive oil, vinegar in a food processor.

2.   Take a large salad bowl and add spinach leaves, toss well with the dressing.

3.   Add remaining ingredients and toss again, season with sunflower seeds and pepper and enjoy!

Nutrition (Per Serving)

Calories: 126

Fat: 10g

Carbohydrates: 10g

Protein: 2g

Elegant Corn Salad

Serving: 6

Prep Time: 10 minutes

Cooking Time: 2 hours

Ingredients:

2 ounces prosciutto, cut into strips

1 teaspoon olive oil

2 cups corn

1/2 cup salt-free tomato sauce

1 teaspoon garlic, minced

1 green bell pepper, chopped

How To:

1. Grease your Slow Cooker with oil.

2.   Add corn, prosciutto, garlic, tomato sauce, bell pepper to your Slow Cooker.

3.   Stir and place lid.

4.   Cook on HIGH for 2 hours.

5.   Divide between serving platters and enjoy!

Nutrition (Per Serving)

Calories: 109

Fat: 2g

Carbohydrates: 10g

Protein: 5g

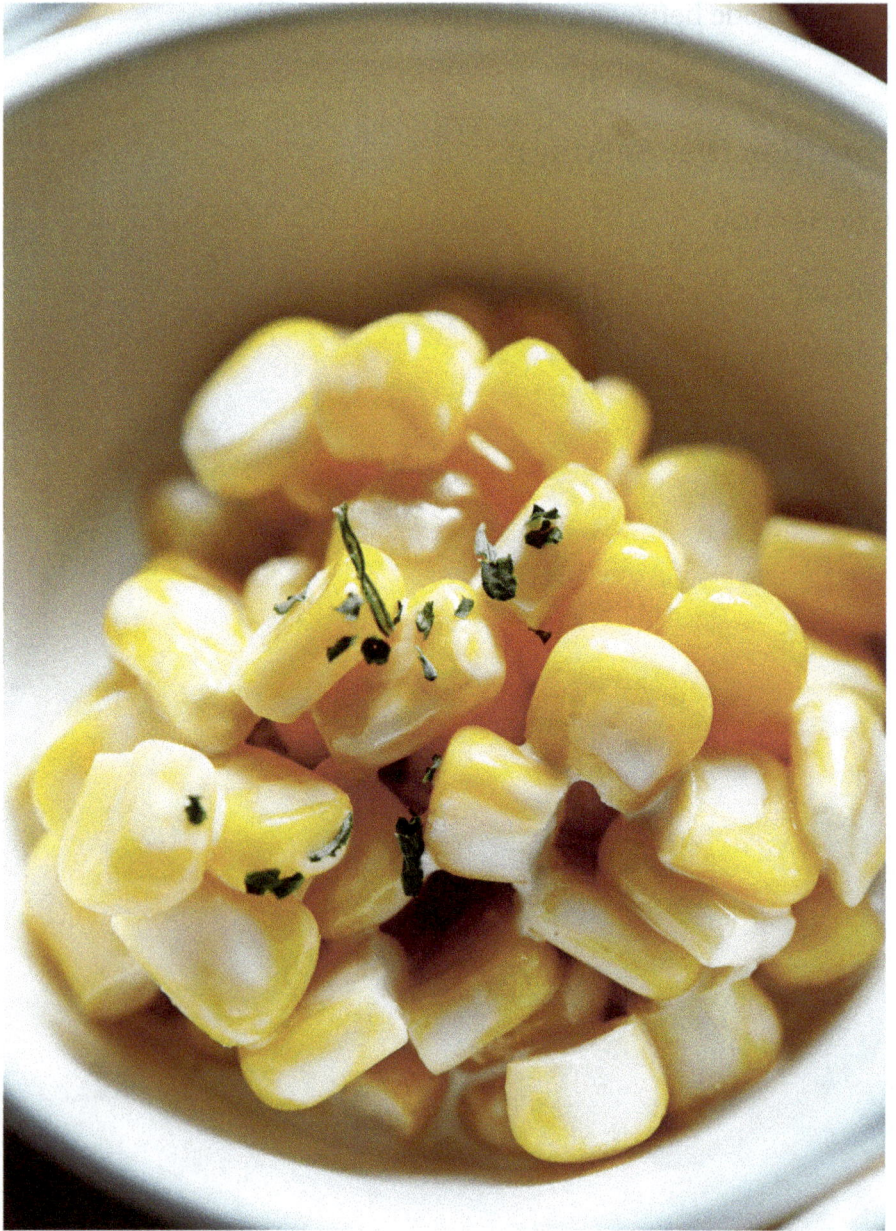

Arabic Fattoush Salad

Serving: 4

Prep Time: 15 minutes

Cook Time: 2-3 minutes

Ingredients:

1 whole wheat pita bread

1 large English cucumber, diced

2 cup grape tomatoes, halved

½ medium red onion, finely diced

¾ cup fresh parsley, chopped

¾ cup mint leaves, chopped

1 clove garlic, minced

¼ cup fat free feta cheese, crumbled

1 tablespoon olive oil

1 teaspoon ground sumac

Juice from ½ a lemon

Salt and pepper as needed

How To:

1.   Mist pita bread with cooking spray.

2.   Season with salt.

3.   Toast until the breads are crispy.

4.   Take a large bowl and add the remaining ingredients and mix (except feta).

5.   Top the mix with diced toasted pita and feta.

6.   Serve and enjoy!

Nutrition (Per Serving)

Calories: 86

Fat: 3g

Carbohydrates: 9g

Protein: 9g

Heart Warming Cauliflower Salad

Serving: 3

Prep Time: 8 minutes

Cook Time: nil

Ingredients:

1 head cauliflower, broken into florets

1 small onion, chopped

1/8 cup extra virgin olive oil

¼ cup apple cider vinegar

½ teaspoon of sea salt

½ teaspoon of black pepper

¼ cup dried cranberries

¼ cup pumpkin seeds

How To:

1.   Wash the cauliflower and break it up into small florets.

2.   Transfer to a bowl.

3.   Whisk oil, vinegar, salt and pepper in another bowl.

4.   Add pumpkin seeds, cranberries to the bowl with dressing.

5.   Mix well and pour the dressing over the cauliflower.

6.   Add onions and toss.

7.   Chill and serve.

8.   Enjoy!

Nutrition (Per Serving)

Calories: 163

Fat: 11g

Carbohydrates: 16g

Protein: 3g

Great Greek Sardine Salad

Serving: 2

Prep Time: 10 minutes

Cook Time: 10 minutes

Ingredients:

2 tablespoons extra virgin olive oil

1 garlic clove, minced

2 teaspoons dried oregano

½ teaspoon freshly ground pepper

3 medium tomatoes, cut into large sized chunks

1 can (15 ounces) rinsed chickpeas

1/3 cup feta cheese, crumbled

¼ cup red onion, sliced

2 tablespoons Kalamata olives, sliced

2 cans 4-ounce drained sardines, with bones and packed in either oil or water

How To:

1.   Take a large bowl and whisk in lemon juice, oregano, garlic, oil, pepper and mix well.

2.   Add tomatoes, chickpeas, cucumber, olives, feta and mix.

3.   Divide the salad amongst serving platter and top with sardines.

4.   Enjoy!

Nutrition (Per Serving)

Calories: 347

Fat: 18g

Carbohydrates: 29g

Protein: 17g

Shrimp and Egg Medley

Serving: 4

Prep Time: 15 minutes

Cook Time: nil

Ingredients:

4 hard-boiled eggs, peeled and chopped

1-pound cooked shrimp, peeled and deveined, chopped

1 sprig fresh dill, chopped

¼ cup mayonnaise

1 teaspoon Dijon mustard

4 fresh lettuce leaves

How To:

1.   Take a large serving bowl and add the listed ingredients (except lettuce).

2.   Stir well.

3.   Serve over bed of lettuce leaves.

4.   Enjoy!

Nutrition (Per Serving)

Calories: 292

Fat: 17g

Carbohydrates: 1.6g

Protein: 30g

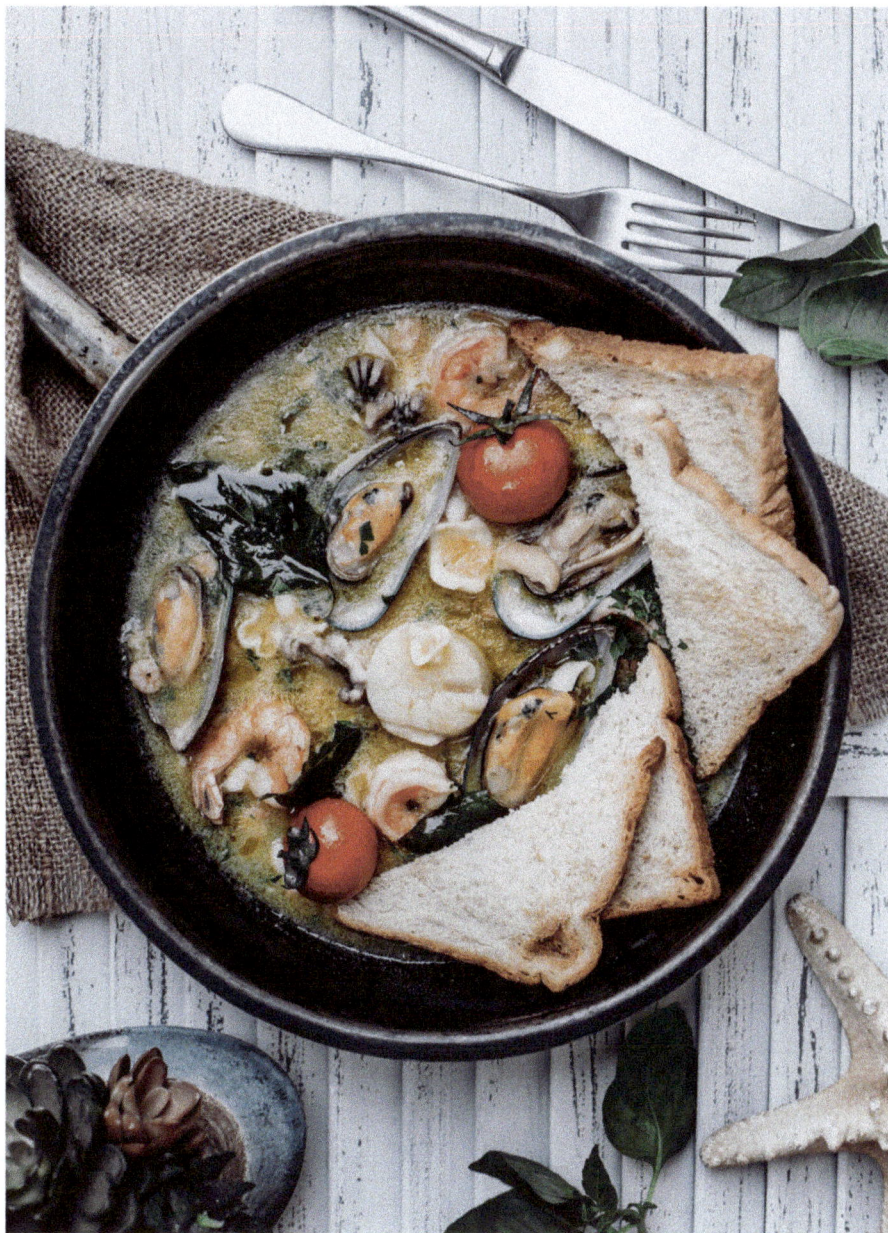

www.ingramcontent.com/pod-product-compliance
Lightning Source LLC
Chambersburg PA
CBHW050750030426
42336CB00012B/1755